I0449521

MicNic Editions

Gratitude Journal

Mickaël Nicotera

This books belongs to

....

Date ...... / ...... / ......

CHALLENGE OF THE WEEK
Call an old friend...

I am very proud of...

1. ....
2. ....
3. ....

What would really make me happy today...

1. ....
2. ....
3. ....

Three surprising things that have happened...

1. ....
2. ....
3. ....

Date ...... / ...... / ......

CHALLENGE OF THE WEEK
Eat your favourite meal

I am very proud of...

1. ....

2. ....

3. ....

What would really make me happy today...

1. ....

2. ....

3. ....

Three surprising things that have happened...

1. ....

2. ....

3. ....

Date ...... / ...... / ......

CHALLENGE OF THE WEEK

Sing in the shower

I am very proud of...

1. ....
2. ....
3. ....

What would really make me happy today...

1. ....
2. ....
3. ....

Three surprising things that have happened...

1. ....
2. ....
3. ....

Date ...... / ...... / ......

CHALLENGE OF THE WEEK

Talk to a stranger

I am very proud of...

1. ....
2. ....
3. ....

What would really make me happy today...

1. ....
2. ....
3. ....

Three surprising things that have happened...

1. ....
2. ....
3. ....

Date ...... / ...... / ......

CHALLENGE OF THE WEEK
Buy yourself a gift

I am very proud of...

1. ....
2. ....
3. ....

What would really make me happy today...

1. ....
2. ....
3. ....

Three surprising things that have happened...

1. ....
2. ....
3. ....

Date ...... / ...... / ......

CHALLENGE OF THE WEEK

Tell someone you love him

I am very proud of...

1. ....
2. ....
3. ....

What would really make me happy today...

1. ....
2. ....
3. ....

Three surprising things that have happened...

1. ....
2. ....
3. ....

Date ...... / ...... / ......

CHALLENGE OF THE WEEK
Look through old pictures

I am very proud of...

1. ....

2. ....

3. ....

What would really make me happy today...

1. ....

2. ....

3. ....

Three surprising things that have happened...

1. ....

2. ....

3. ....

Date ...... / ...... / ......

CHALLENGE OF THE WEEK

Jogging

I am very proud of...

1. ....
2. ....
3. ....

What would really make me happy today...

1. ....
2. ....
3. ....

Three surprising things that have happened...

1. ....
2. ....
3. ....

Date ...... / ...... / ......

CHALLENGE OF THE WEEK

Leave your mobile phone at home for one day

I am very proud of...

1. ....

2. ....

3. ....

What would really make me happy today...

1. ....

2. ....

3. ....

Three surprising things that have happened...

1. ....

2. ....

3. ....

Date ...... / ...... / ......

CHALLENGE OF THE WEEK

Buy someone a drink

I am very proud of...

1. ....

2. ....

3. ....

What would really make me happy today...

1. ....

2. ....

3. ....

Three surprising things that have happened...

1. ....

2. ....

3. ....

Date ...... / ...... / ......

CHALLENGE OF THE WEEK
Dance

I am very proud of...

1. ....
2. ....
3. ....

What would really make me happy today...

1. ....
2. ....
3. ....

Three surprising things that have happened...

1. ....
2. ....
3. ....

Date ...... / ...... / ......

CHALLENGE OF THE WEEK

Walk in a park

I am very proud of...

1. ....
2. ....
3. ....

What would really make me happy today...

1. ....
2. ....
3. ....

Three surprising things that have happened...

1. ....
2. ....
3. ....

Date ...... / ...... / ......

CHALLENGE OF THE WEEK

Take a relaxing bath

I am very proud of...

1. ....

2. ....

3. ....

What would really make me happy today...

1. ....

2. ....

3. ....

Three surprising things that have happened...

1. ....

2. ....

3. ....

Date .... / .... / ....

CHALLENGE OF THE WEEK

Buy a coffee for a homeless person

I am very proud of...

1. ....

2. ....

3. ....

What would really make me happy today...

1. ....

2. ....

3. ....

Three surprising things that have happened...

1. ....

2. ....

3. ....

Date ...... / ...... / ......

CHALLENGE OF THE WEEK

Smile with strangers

I am very proud of...

1. ....
2. ....
3. ....

What would really make me happy today...

1. ....
2. ....
3. ....

Three surprising things that have happened...

1. ....
2. ....
3. ....

Date ...... / ...... / ......

CHALLENGE OF THE WEEK

Watch your favorite movie

I am very proud of...

1. ....

2. ....

3. ....

What would really make me happy today...

1. ....

2. ....

3. ....

Three surprising things that have happened...

1. ....

2. ....

3. ....

Date ...... / ...... / ......

CHALLENGE OF THE WEEK
Buy yourself a new cloth

I am very proud of...

1. ....
2. ....
3. ....

What would really make me happy today...

1. ....
2. ....
3. ....

Three surprising things that have happened...

1. ....
2. ....
3. ....

Date ...... / ...... / ......

CHALLENGE OF THE WEEK

Eat a chocolate bar

I am very proud of...

1. ....

2. ....

3. ....

What would really make me happy today...

1. ....

2. ....

3. ....

Three surprising things that have happened...

1. ....

2. ....

3. ....

Date ...... / ...... / ......

CHALLENGE OF THE WEEK

Brush your teeth with your left hand

I am very proud of...

1. ....
2. ....
3. ....

What would really make me happy today...

1. ....
2. ....
3. ....

Three surprising things that have happened...

1. ....
2. ....
3. ....

Date ...... / ...... / ......

CHALLENGE OF THE WEEK
Wash windows

I am very proud of...

1. ....
2. ....
3. ....

What would really make me happy today...

1. ....
2. ....
3. ....

Three surprising things that have happened...

1. ....
2. ....
3. ....

Date ...... / ...... / ......

CHALLENGE OF THE WEEK

Cook a delicious cake

I am very proud of...

1. ....

2. ....

3. ....

What would really make me happy today...

1. ....

2. ....

3. ....

Three surprising things that have happened...

1. ....

2. ....

3. ....

Date ...... / ...... / ......

CHALLENGE OF THE WEEK

Have a rest

I am very proud of...

1. ....

2. ....

3. ....

What would really make me happy today...

1. ....

2. ....

3. ....

Three surprising things that have happened...

1. ....

2. ....

3. ....

Date ...... / ...... / ......

CHALLENGE OF THE WEEK

Read a chapter of a book

I am very proud of...

1. ....
2. ....
3. ....

What would really make me happy today...

1. ....
2. ....
3. ....

Three surprising things that have happened...

1. ....
2. ....
3. ....

Date ...... / ...... / ......

CHALLENGE OF THE WEEK

Buy yourself new shoes

I am very proud of...

1. ....

2. ....

3. ....

What would really make me happy today...

1. ....

2. ....

3. ....

Three surprising things that have happened...

1. ....

2. ....

3. ....

Date ...... / ...... / ......

CHALLENGE OF THE WEEK

Eat a burger

I am very proud of...

1. ....
2. ....
3. ....

What would really make me happy today...

1. ....
2. ....
3. ....

Three surprising things that have happened...

1. ....
2. ....
3. ....

Date ...... / ...... / ......

CHALLENGE OF THE WEEK

Watch a bird

I am very proud of...

1. ....
2. ....
3. ....

What would really make me happy today...

1. ....
2. ....
3. ....

Three surprising things that have happened...

1. ....
2. ....
3. ....

Date ...... / ...... / ......

CHALLENGE OF THE WEEK

Watch a movie, eating popcorn

I am very proud of...

1. ....

2. ....

3. ....

What would really make me happy today...

1. ....

2. ....

3. ....

Three surprising things that have happened...

1. ....

2. ....

3. ....

Date ...... / ...... / ......

CHALLENGE OF THE WEEK

Write a poem

I am very proud of...

1. ....
2. ....
3. ....

What would really make me happy today...

1. ....
2. ....
3. ....

Three surprising things that have happened...

1. ....
2. ....
3. ....

Date ...... / ...... / ......

CHALLENGE OF THE WEEK

Cook for someone you love

I am very proud of...

1. ....

2. ....

3. ....

What would really make me happy today...

1. ....

2. ....

3. ....

Three surprising things that have happened...

1. ....

2. ....

3. ....

Date ...... / ...... / ......

CHALLENGE OF THE WEEK

Pick a bouquet of flowers

I am very proud of...

1. ....

2. ....

3. ....

What would really make me happy today...

1. ....

2. ....

3. ....

Three surprising things that have happened...

1. ....

2. ....

3. ....

Date ...... / ...... / ......

CHALLENGE OF THE WEEK
Find your next holiday destination

I am very proud of...

1. ....
2. ....
3. ....

What would really make me happy today...

1. ....
2. ....
3. ....

Three surprising things that have happened...

1. ....
2. ....
3. ....

Date ...... / ...... / ......

CHALLENGE OF THE WEEK

Make pancakes

I am very proud of...

1. ....
2. ....
3. ....

What would really make me happy today...

1. ....
2. ....
3. ....

Three surprising things that have happened...

1. ....
2. ....
3. ....

Date ...... / ...... / ......

CHALLENGE OF THE WEEK

Spend a day under the duvet

I am very proud of...

1. ....

2. ....

3. ....

What would really make me happy today...

1. ....

2. ....

3. ....

Three surprising things that have happened...

1. ....

2. ....

3. ....

Date ...... / ...... / ......

CHALLENGE OF THE WEEK

Do not eat any meat for three days

I am very proud of...

1. ....
2. ....
3. ....

What would really make me happy today...

1. ....
2. ....
3. ....

Three surprising things that have happened...

1. ....
2. ....
3. ....

Date ....../....../......

CHALLENGE OF THE WEEK

Give a gift to someone

I am very proud of...

1. ....
2. ....
3. ....

What would really make me happy today...

1. ....
2. ....
3. ....

Three surprising things that have happened...

1. ....
2. ....
3. ....

Date ...... / ...... / ......

CHALLENGE OF THE WEEK

Put in order your desktop

I am very proud of...

1. ....

2. ....

3. ....

What would really make me happy today...

1. ....

2. ....

3. ....

Three surprising things that have happened...

1. ....

2. ....

3. ....

Date ...... / ...... / ......

CHALLENGE OF THE WEEK

Watch a hilarious video on the Internet

I am very proud of...

1. ....
2. ....
3. ....

What would really make me happy today...

1. ....
2. ....
3. ....

Three surprising things that have happened...

1. ....
2. ....
3. ....

Date ...... / ...... / ......

CHALLENGE OF THE WEEK

Make a picnic lunch

I am very proud of...

1. ....

2. ....

3. ....

What would really make me happy today...

1. ....

2. ....

3. ....

Three surprising things that have happened...

1. ....

2. ....

3. ....

Date ...... / ...... / ......

CHALLENGE OF THE WEEK

Germinate a bean seed

I am very proud of...

1. ....

2. ....

3. ....

What would really make me happy today...

1. ....

2. ....

3. ....

Three surprising things that have happened...

1. ....

2. ....

3. ....

Date ...... / ...... / ......

CHALLENGE OF THE WEEK
Go to the restaurant

I am very proud of...

1. ....
2. ....
3. ....

What would really make me happy today...

1. ....
2. ....
3. ....

Three surprising things that have happened...

1. ....
2. ....
3. ....

Date ...... / ...... / ......

CHALLENGE OF THE WEEK

Say Yes to everything for a day

I am very proud of...

1. ....
2. ....
3. ....

What would really make me happy today...

1. ....
2. ....
3. ....

Three surprising things that have happened...

1. ....
2. ....
3. ....

Date ...... / ...... / ......

CHALLENGE OF THE WEEK

Eat Brussels sprouts

I am very proud of...

1. ....

2. ....

3. ....

What would really make me happy today...

1. ....

2. ....

3. ....

Three surprising things that have happened...

1. ....

2. ....

3. ....

Date ...... / ...... / ......

CHALLENGE OF THE WEEK

Learn three new french words

I am very proud of...

1. ....
2. ....
3. ....

What would really make me happy today...

1. ....
2. ....
3. ....

Three surprising things that have happened...

1. ....
2. ....
3. ....

Date ...... / ...... / ......

CHALLENGE OF THE WEEK
Learn a new yoga pose

I am very proud of...

1. ....
2. ....
3. ....

What would really make me happy today...

1. ....
2. ....
3. ....

Three surprising things that have happened...

1. ....
2. ....
3. ....

Date ...... / ...... / ......

CHALLENGE OF THE WEEK
Laugh

I am very proud of...

1. ....

2. ....

3. ....

What would really make me happy today...

1. ....

2. ....

3. ....

Three surprising things that have happened...

1. ....

2. ....

3. ....

Date ...... / ...... / ......

CHALLENGE OF THE WEEK

Only drink water over the entire week

I am very proud of...

1. ....
2. ....
3. ....

What would really make me happy today...

1. ....
2. ....
3. ....

Three surprising things that have happened...

1. ....
2. ....
3. ....

Date ...... / ...... / ......

CHALLENGE OF THE WEEK

Admire a sunset

I am very proud of...

1. ....
2. ....
3. ....

What would really make me happy today...

1. ....
2. ....
3. ....

Three surprising things that have happened...

1. ....
2. ....
3. ....

Date ...... / ...... / ......

CHALLENGE OF THE WEEK

Hug someone

I am very proud of...

1. ....

2. ....

3. ....

What would really make me happy today...

1. ....

2. ....

3. ....

Three surprising things that have happened...

1. ....

2. ....

3. ....

Date ...... / ...... / ......

CHALLENGE OF THE WEEK
Buy yourself jewelry

I am very proud of...

1. ....

2. ....

3. ....

What would really make me happy today...

1. ....

2. ....

3. ....

Three surprising things that have happened...

1. ....

2. ....

3. ....

Date ...... / ...... / ......

CHALLENGE OF THE WEEK
Watch a childhood cartoon

I am very proud of...

1. ....

2. ....

3. ....

What would really make me happy today...

1. ....

2. ....

3. ....

Three surprising things that have happened...

1. ....

2. ....

3. ....

Date ...... / ...... / ......

CHALLENGE OF THE WEEK

Wear very colorful clothing for a day

I am very proud of...

1. ....
2. ....
3. ....

What would really make me happy today...

1. ....
2. ....
3. ....

Three surprising things that have happened...

1. ....
2. ....
3. ....

Date ...... / ...... / ......

CHALLENGE OF THE WEEK

Do a bike tour

I am very proud of...

1. ....

2. ....

3. ....

What would really make me happy today...

1. ....

2. ....

3. ....

Three surprising things that have happened...

1. ....

2. ....

3. ....

Date ...... / ...... / ......

CHALLENGE OF THE WEEK

Eat an unknown fruit

I am very proud of...

1. ....
2. ....
3. ....

What would really make me happy today...

1. ....
2. ....
3. ....

Three surprising things that have happened...

1. ....
2. ....
3. ....

Printed by Lulu.com
January 2016
N° ISBN : 978-1-326-54872-8

www.ingramcontent.com/pod-product-compliance
Lightning Source LLC
Chambersburg PA
CBHW070334290526
45791CB00003B/1326